Contents

Profile of Dr J Gordon Gadsby

Ph.D BA(Hons) RGN RMN DipN(Lond) MISBM DHP DHS

Dr J Gordon Gadsby is a leading clinical specialist in neuro-electric acupuncture and transcutaneous electrical nerve stimulation. He now practices in the private health care sector, following a successful twenty eight year career in psychiatric and general NHS hospital nursing.

He has practised in Leicester for the last twenty years as an electro-acupuncturist, neuro-electric acupuncturist and TENS specialist. He has a BA(Hons) degree in Health Studies and a doctorate in electroanalgesia from the De Montfort University, Leicester. Gordon's Ph.D researched the historical and contemporary developments of electrical treatment of chronic and low-back pain, using transcutaneous electrical nerve stimulation (TENS) and acupuncture-like TENS, within the framework of the Cochrane Collaboration.

Gordon was appointed as a consultant to Body Clock Health Care Limited in December 1995 to advise on therapeutic applications, research and new product information.

For more information on Dr Gordon Gadsby visit his Internet Website on:
http://freespace.virgin.net/joseph.gadsby/index.htm

I. Introduction - What is TENS all about?

TENS stands for Transcutaneous Electrical Nerve Stimulation. The treatment consists of passing mild electrical impulses through your skin into the nerve fibres which lie below. Contact is made with your skin via electrodes. TENS electrodes are generally placed around the painful area, over the painful area or over acupuncture points.

TENS impulses help your body produce its own pain killing substances. A TENS unit does not provide a direct cure for the problems responsible for your pain, but it alleviates your pain sensation. It also stimulates various anti-inflammatory substances, which help your body with the healing process. There are two generally accepted theories on how TENS works:

a: The Gate Control Theory

The TENS message is carried to the spinal cord faster than a pain message and closes a hypothetical gate, inhibiting the pain message to the brain. This TENS treatment is also known as "conventional" or "high frequency" and applies when the Pulse Rate is set at 60-80 pulses per second or more. The sensation produced with this setting can be described as a steady "buzzing" or "tingling" feeling. Many find high frequency TENS produces the quickest pain relief, often with several hours of relief, after a treatment of one hour.

b: Acupuncture-like TENS or low frequency TENS

Acupuncture-like TENS or low frequency TENS stimulates the body to release endorphins, the body's own pain killing substances. This applies when the Pulse Rate setting is below 4 pulses per second - and usually at 2 pulses per second. These low frequency treatments are adjusted to an intensity that produces slight muscle twitching and are described as "tapping" or "pulsating". Patients find this type of treatment takes longer, at least 20-30 minutes to be effective, but the result of a 30-60 minute treatment can last for a much longer period; hours and sometimes days.

The degree of pain relief varies from person to person and it is difficult to predict just how effective TENS will be until you try it. The best results are obtained by selecting the most appropriate electrode position and frequency settings for your particular pain.

A brief history of electrotherapy and TENS

Although in its present form TENS is of relatively recent origin, therapeutic electrical stimulation of the human body has been employed in various forms since early times. Stone carvings from the Egyptian Fifth Dynasty made in approximately 2500BC show an electric fish being used to treat pain. In AD46 the Roman physician, Scribonious Largus recorded the introduction of the electrical powers of the fish into clinical medicine as a cure for headache and gout. In some parts of the world, the electric catfish and electric rays continued to be used for the treatment of pain and other conditions up until the end of the nineteenth century. Electrostimulation, using static electrical machines, came into prominence in the mid eighteenth century and continued in popularity through the eighteenth and nineteenth centuries. However, it fell out of favour in the early part of the twentieth century due to the availability of a wider range of analgesic drugs.

The present day use of TENS began after the 1965 publication of a landmark paper by Melzack and Wall entitled "Pain Mechanisms: A New Theory". Its use is expanding from pain clinics to emergency departments, operating theatres, labour wards, surgeries and self care.

What conditions can be treated with TENS?

Many painful conditions (and some non-painful conditions) can be treated with TENS. As with all other forms of therapy, it is essential to have the cause of your pain diagnosed by your medical adviser beforehand. Pain can be a warning sign, to alert us that something may be wrong. However, some types of chronic pain appear to be of no real value and may result in continuous discomfort, depression, restriction in our movements and general functioning. Acute pain is usually more severe and of shorter duration, e.g childbirth, trauma or surgery. Acute and chronic pain can be treated with TENS and some of the more common examples are listed below.

- Rheumatoid arthritis
- Osteoarthritis of one or several joints
- Ankylosing spondylosis
- Neck pain, cervical spondylosis, whiplash injuries
- Low back pain resulting from strains, prolapsed disc, spondylitis,
- Osteoporosis
- Referred pains such as sciatica
- Fibrositis/myofascial pain syndromes
- Acute sprains/strains e.g sports and occupational injuries
- Tendonitis/bursitis
- Carpal tunnel syndrome
- Migraine and headaches
- Peripheral nerve injuries and neuropathy of various causes
- Phantom limb pain
- Post herpetic (shingles) neuralgia
- Post operative neuralgia and scar tissue pain
- Pain in cancer and the terminally ill
- Labour pain
- Nausea and vomiting
- Stress and Insomnia
- Numerous other pain conditions

However, it may be dangerous to mask pain associated with an unknown illness or a recent uninvestigated injury. You should check with your health care adviser for an accurate diagnosis, before using TENS.

Why should I use a Body Clock TENS?

Body Clock offers a wide range of units, which are fully compliant with current medical device regulations. These have been tried and tested over many years by the author and other practitioners. Body Clock only make the highest quality TENS units known for their ease of use and latest technology.

How will TENS help my pain?

The aim of TENS treatment is to promote pain relief, an increase in movement and function of the affected area, and to decrease pain medication. Good results have been obtained over the past twenty-five years in hundreds of studies, surveys and systematic reviews conducted on both acute and chronic pain patients. By the year 2000 there were nearly 500 studies and reviews on electrical stimulation methods recorded in the Cochrane Library database alone, the most important source of high quality medical research in the world today. The extensive Medline database listed more than 800. We can now say that TENS provides useful relief for most people with acute, subacute or chronic pain. In addition TENS is a safe, non invasive treatment, economical and easy to use.

II. Electrode Placement and Charts

The importance of accurate electrode placement

We cannot stress too strongly that correct electrode placement is vital to obtain the best results from your Body Clock TENS. Please see the following charts which have been specially prepared to help you.

The most important aspects of TENS electrode placement is to position them so that the current passes through the painful area, or along the nerves leading from the pain, or over acupuncture points. If your Body Clock TENS is a dual channel unit, with two sets of leads and electrodes, then it is possible to treat two different areas of pain at once.

How to use the electrode placement charts.

Check the index on page 6 for the chart most applicable to your own pain problem. We have selected the easiest and most frequently used electrode placement positions. However there are alternatives, which may be advised by your medical practitioner.

Charts

Page

Key: ■■ = 1st pair of electrodes □□ = 2nd pair of electrodes - If using a dual channel TENS
Electrodes supplied are single colour. Black and white squares are for indicating electrode placement only.

Low back pain chart 1

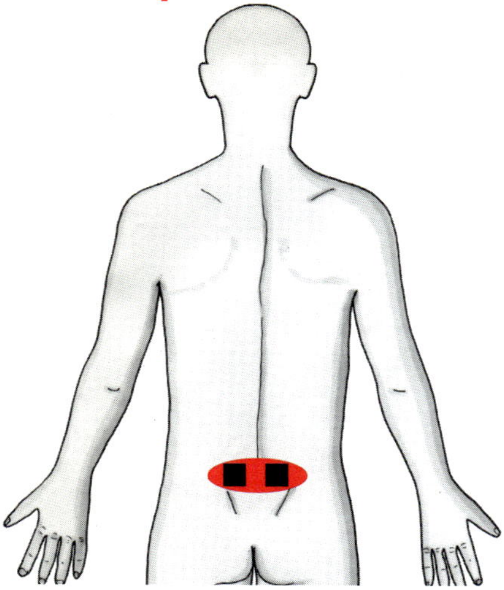

Low Back pain is shown by the red "pain zone". The black squares inside the "pain zone" represent a pair of electrodes. Each electrode is placed on the lower back as shown above.

Low back pain chart 2

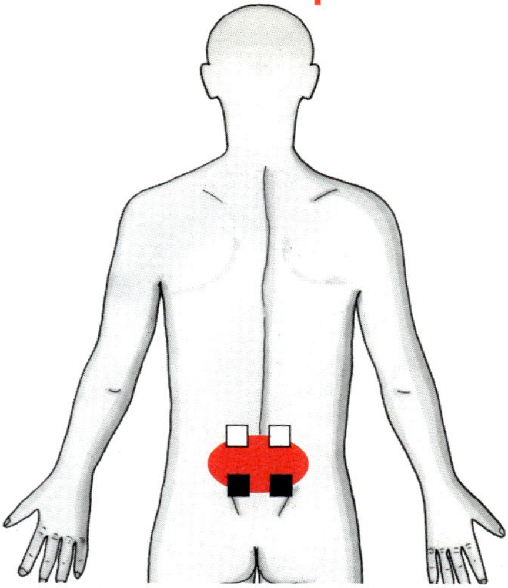

Low Back pain is shown by the red "pain zone". The black and white squares inside the "pain zone" represent two pairs of electrodes, placed on the lower back as shown

Upper back pain chart 1

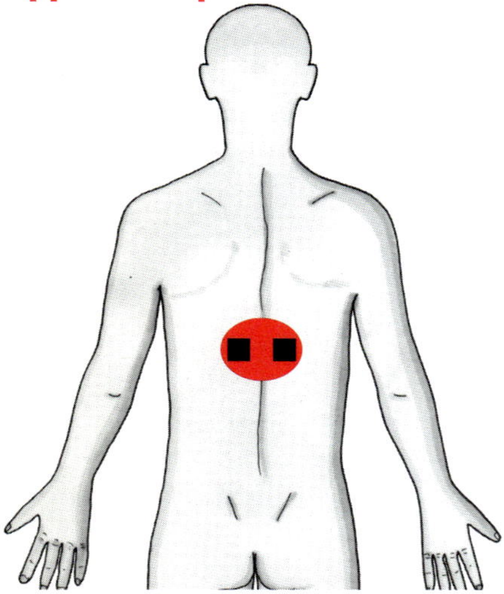

Upper back pain is shown by the red "pain zone". The black squares inside the "pain zone" represent a pair of electrodes. Each electrode is placed on the back as shown above.

Upper back pain chart 2

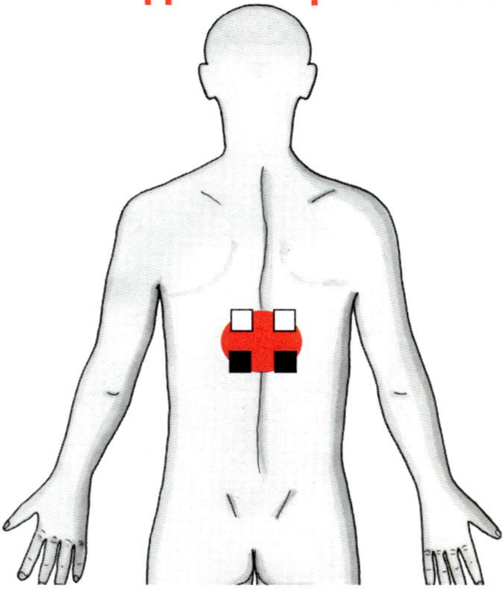

Upper back pain is shown by the red "pain zone". The black and white squares inside the "pain zone" represent two pairs of electrodes, placed on the back as shown above.

Back pain with sciatica chart 1

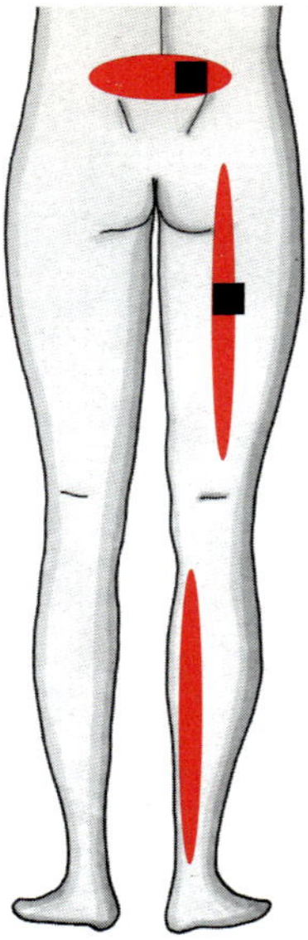

Back pain with Sciatica is shown by the red "pain zone". The black squares inside the "pain zone" represent a pair of electrodes. Each electrode is placed on the body as shown above.

Back pain with sciatica chart 2

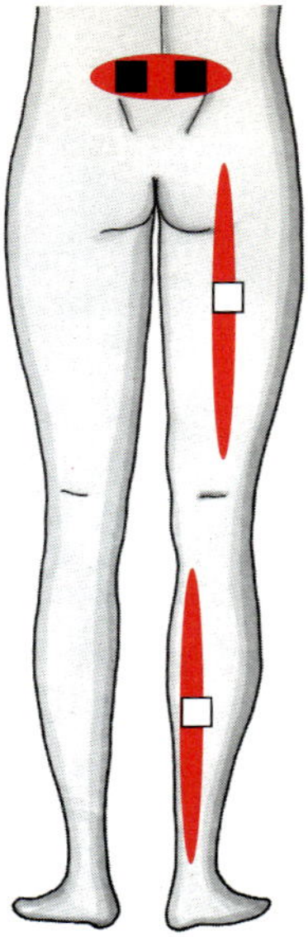

Back pain with sciatica is shown by the red "pain zone". The black and white squares inside the "pain zone" represent two pairs of electrodes. Each electrode is placed on the body as shown above.

Ankylosing Spondylitis

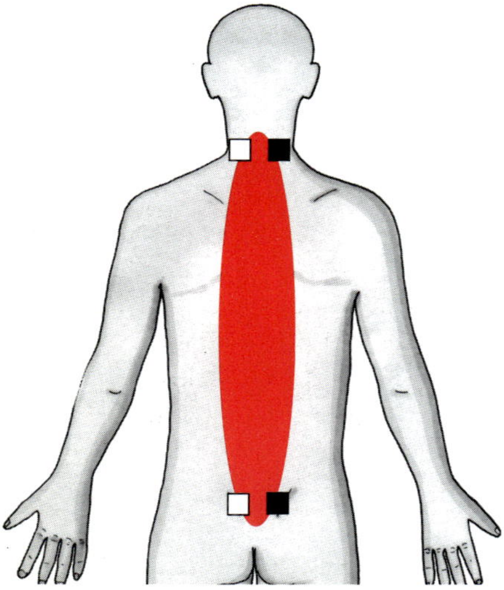

Ankylosing Spondylitis is shown by the red "pain zone". The black and white squares inside the "pain zone" represent two pairs of electrodes. The electrodes are placed on the back as shown in the diagram.

Neck pain and whiplash chart 1

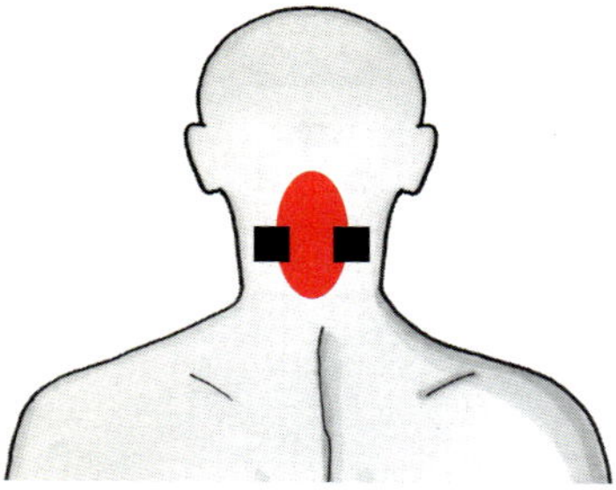

Neck pain/whiplash is shown by the red "pain zone". The black squares inside the "pain zone" represent a pair of electrodes. Each electrode is placed either side of the spine as shown in the diagram to the left.

Neck pain and whiplash chart 2

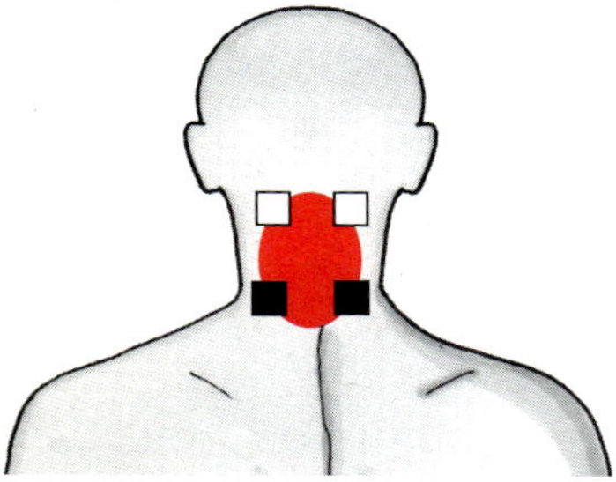

Neck pain/whiplash is shown by the red "pain zone". The black and white squares inside the "pain zone" represent two pairs of electrodes. Each electrode is placed either side of the spine as shown in the diagram to the left.

Shoulder pain and frozen shoulder

Outer aspect of arm   Inner aspect of arm

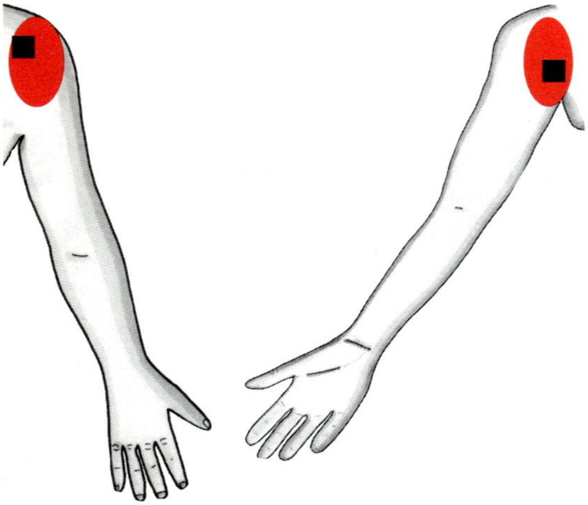

Shoulder pain and frozen shoulder is shown by the red "pain zone". The black squares inside the "pain zone" represent a pair of electrodes. One electrode is placed on the front of the shoulder and the other on the back of the shoulder as shown in the diagrams to the left.

Shoulder pain and frozen shoulder

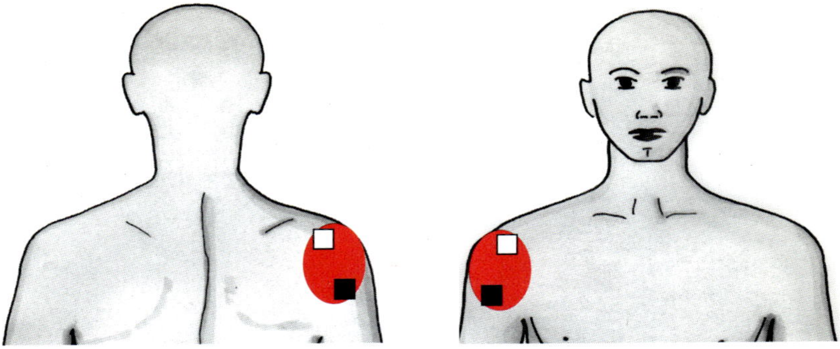

Shoulder pain and frozen shoulder is shown by the red "pain zone" above. The black and white squares inside the "pain zone" represent two pairs of electrodes. Two electrodes are placed on the front of the shoulder and the other two on the back of the shoulder as shown in the diagrams.

Hip pain Chart 1

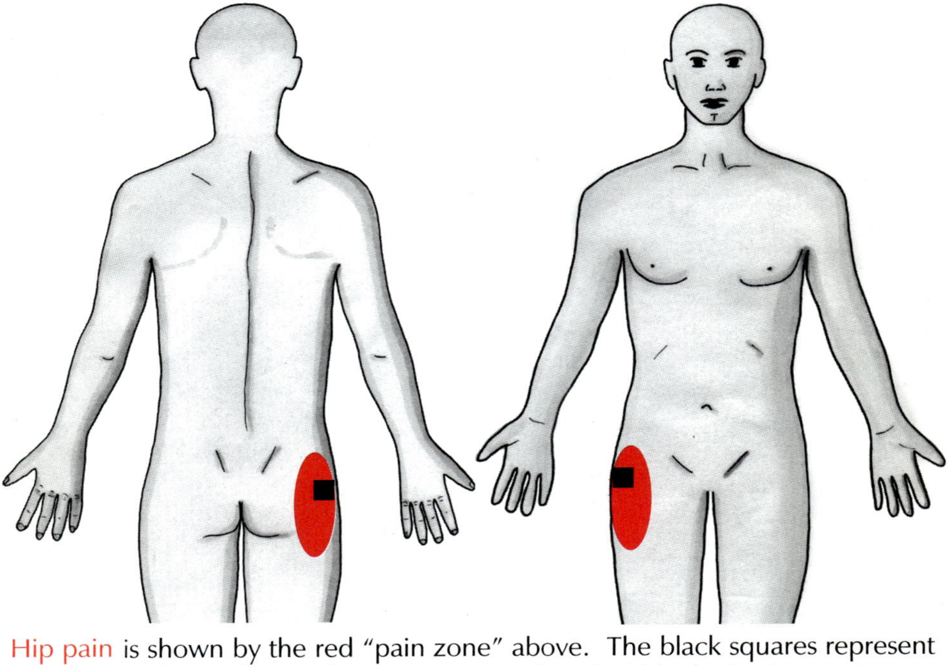

Hip pain is shown by the red "pain zone" above. The black squares represent a set of two electrodes. Both electrodes are placed within the "pain zone" - one at the front and one at the back.

Hip pain Chart 2

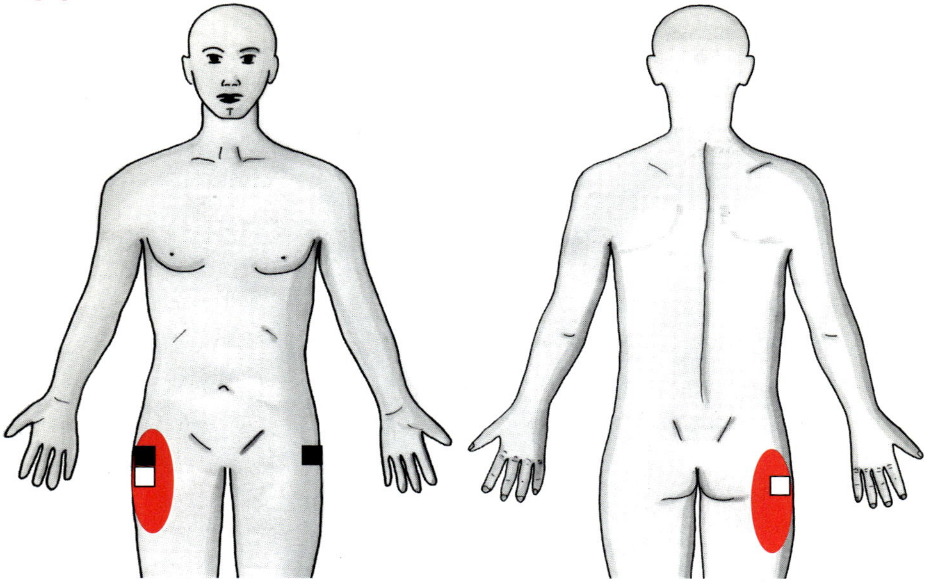

Hip pain is shown by the red "pain zone" above. The black and white squares inside the "pain zone" represent two pairs of electrodes.
a.The white set is placed within the "pain zone" - one at the front and one at the back of the hip.
b.The black set is placed on opposite hips to allow the current to pass straight through the body.

Knee pain Chart 1

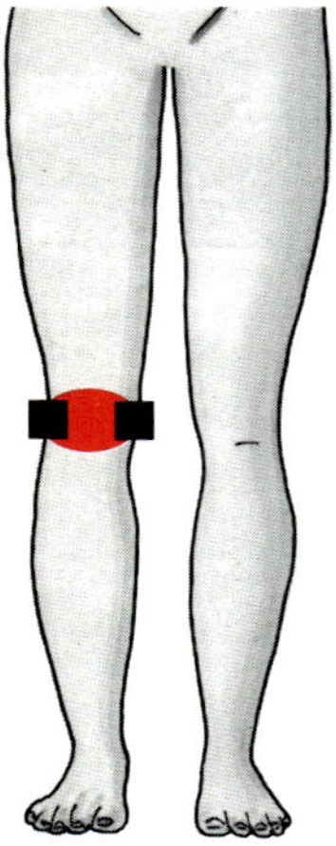

Knee pain is shown by the red "pain zone". The black squares inside the "pain zone" represent a pair of electrodes. These should be placed either side of the knee as shown.

The black and white squares inside the "pain zone" represent two pairs of electrodes. The black electrodes are placed as in chart 1 The white electrodes are placed at the back and front of the knee allowing the current to pass through.

Knee pain Chart 2

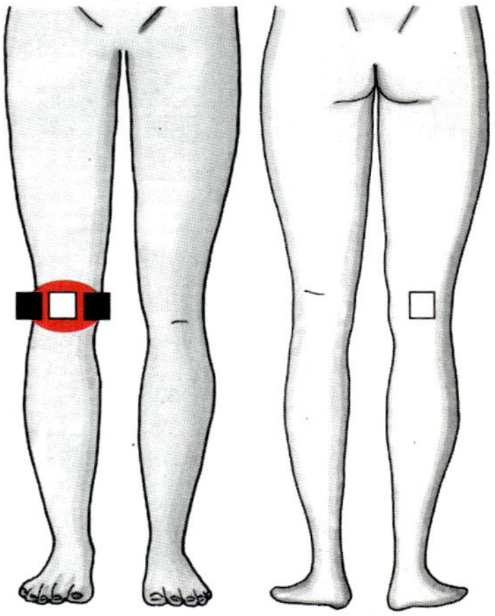

Ankle pain

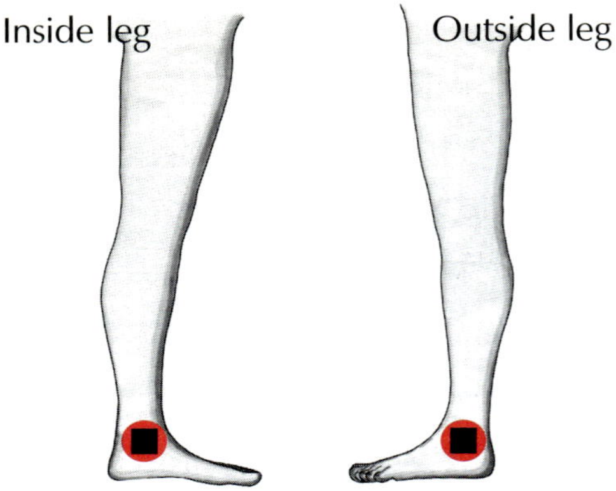

Ankle and foot pain is shown by the red "pain zone". The black squares inside the "pain zone' represent a pair of electrodes. These are placed either side of the ankle as shown in the diagrams to the left.

Achilles tendon pain

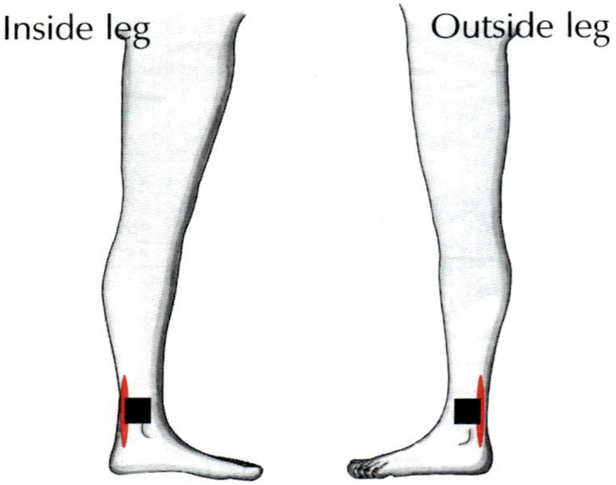

Ankle and foot pain is shown by the red "pain zone". The black squares inside the "pain zone' represent a pair of electrodes. These are placed either side of the leg as shown in the diagrams to the left.

Foot pain

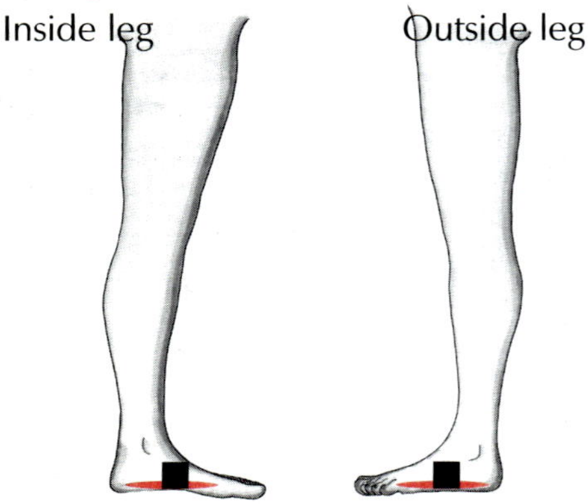

Ankle and foot pain is shown by the red "pain zone". The black squares inside the "pain zone' represent a pair of electrodes. These are placed either side of the foot as shown in the diagrams, or one on the sole and one on the top of the foot.

Phantom limb pain below the knee

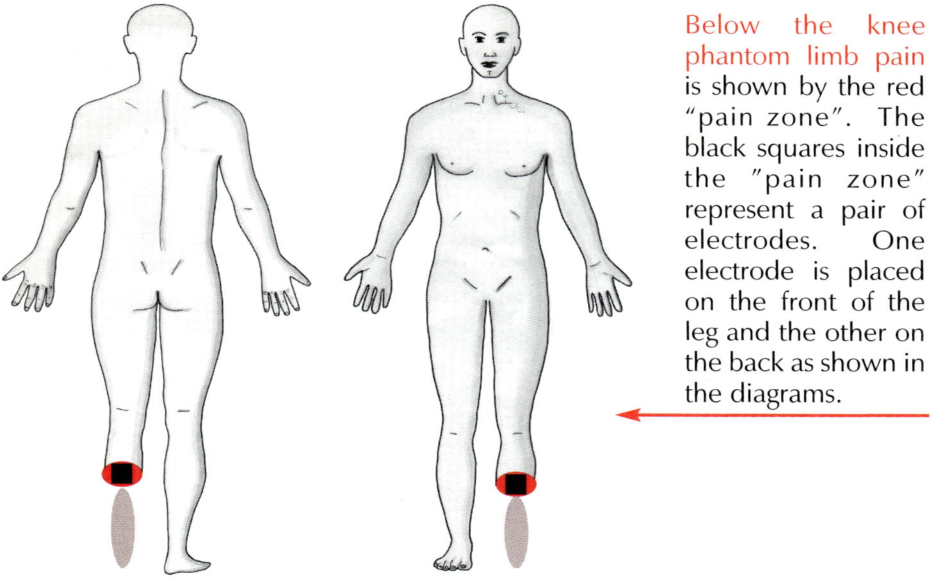

Below the knee phantom limb pain is shown by the red "pain zone". The black squares inside the "pain zone" represent a pair of electrodes. One electrode is placed on the front of the leg and the other on the back as shown in the diagrams.

Phantom limb pain above the knee

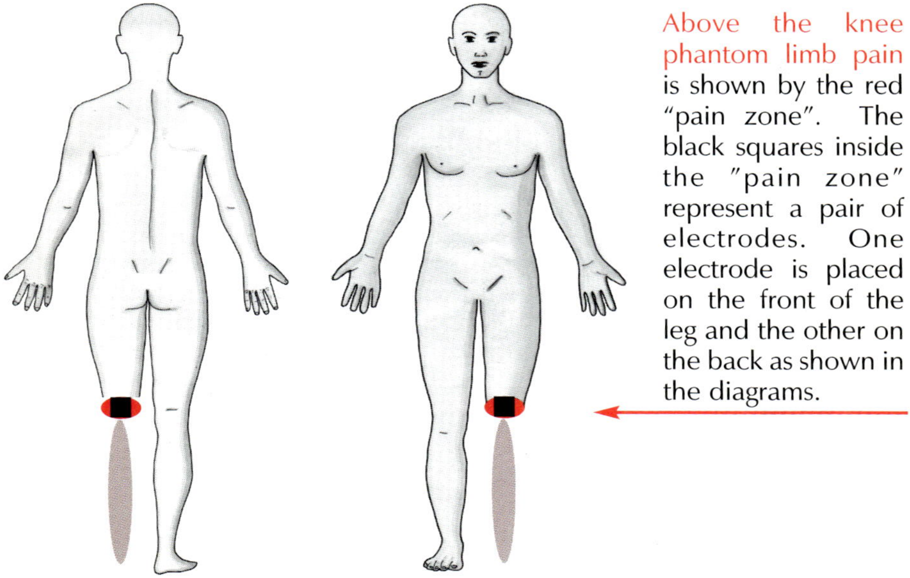

Above the knee phantom limb pain is shown by the red "pain zone". The black squares inside the "pain zone" represent a pair of electrodes. One electrode is placed on the front of the leg and the other on the back as shown in the diagrams.

Phantom limb pain above the knee

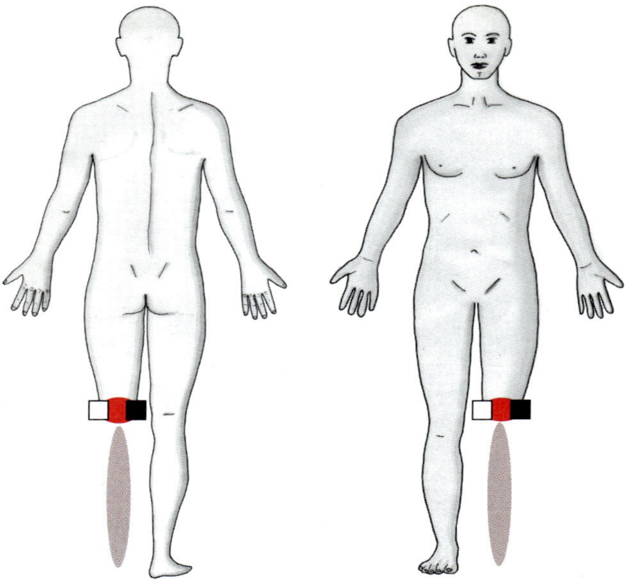

Above the knee phantom limb pain is shown by the red "pain zone". The black and white squares inside the "pain zone" represent two pairs of electrodes. Two electrodes are placed on the front of the leg and the other two on the back of the leg as shown in the diagrams.

Tennis elbow

Outer aspect of arm

Inner aspect of arm

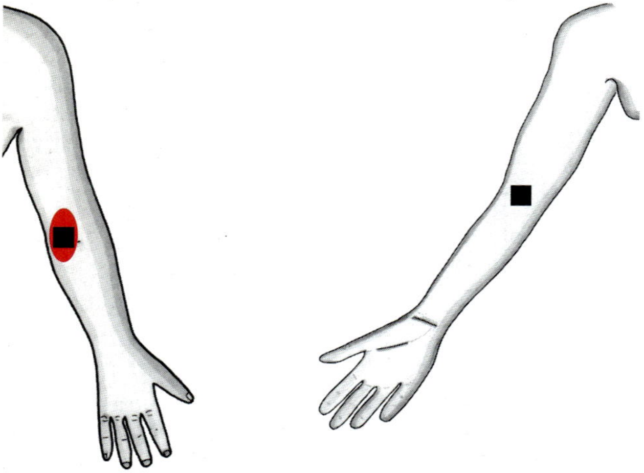

Tennis elbow pain is shown by the red "pain zone". The black squares inside the "pain zone" represent a pair of electrodes. One electrode is placed over the area of pain and the other on the inner aspect of the arm allowing the current to pass through the arm.

Golfers elbow

Outer aspect of arm — Inner aspect of arm

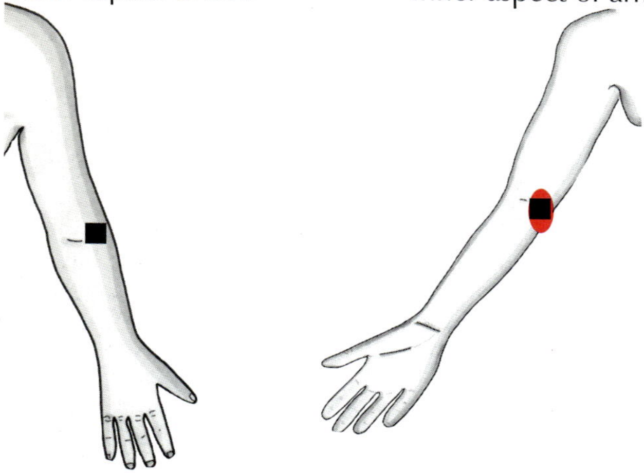

Golfers elbow pain is shown by the red "pain zone". The black squares inside the "pain zone" represent a pair of electrodes. One electrode is placed over the area of pain and the other on the outer aspect of the arm allowing the current to pass through the arm.

Wrist and carpal tunnel syndrome

Outer aspect of arm — Inner aspect of arm

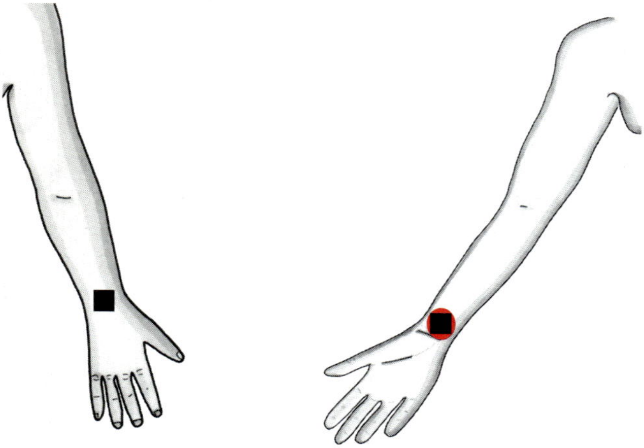

Wrist and carpal tunnel syndrome pain is shown by the red "pain zone". The black squares inside the "pain zone" represent a pair of electrodes. One electrode is placed over the area of pain and the other on the outer aspect of the arm allowing the current to pass through the arm.

Hand and finger pain

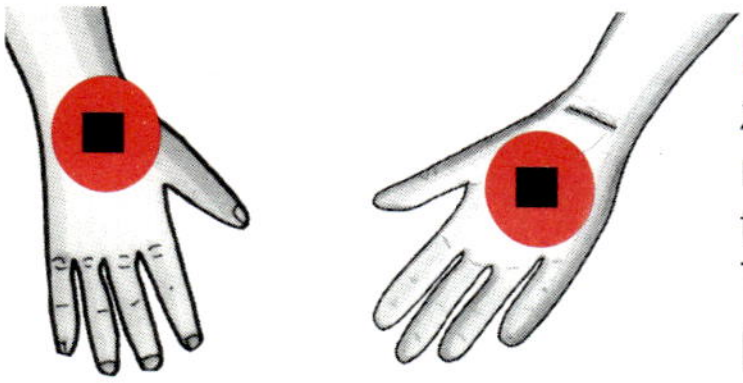

Hand and finger pain is shown by the red "pain zone". The black squares inside the "pain zone" represent a pair of electrodes. These are placed in the pain zone" on opposite sides of the hand. They can also be wrapped around two fingers in pain and secured with tape, if necessary.

Phantom limb pain below the elbow

Outer aspect of arm

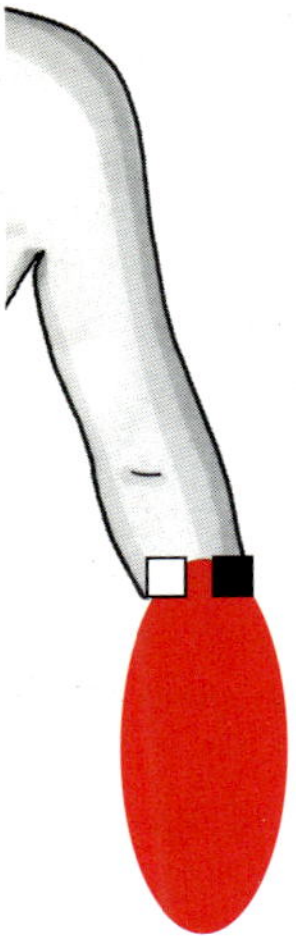

Inner aspect of arm

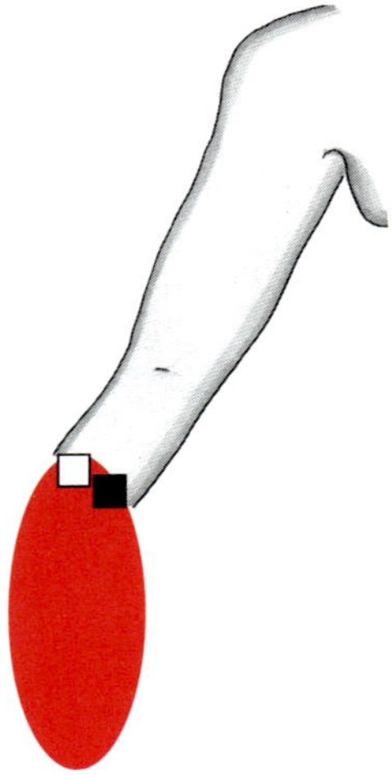

Phantom arm pain - is shown by the red "pain zone". The black and white squares inside the "pain zone" represent two pairs of electrodes. Two electrodes are placed on the front of the arm and the other two on the back as shown in the diagrams. If you are using only one pair of electrodes, apply each pad centrally to the front and back of the stump.

Phantom limb pain above the elbow

Outer aspect of arm

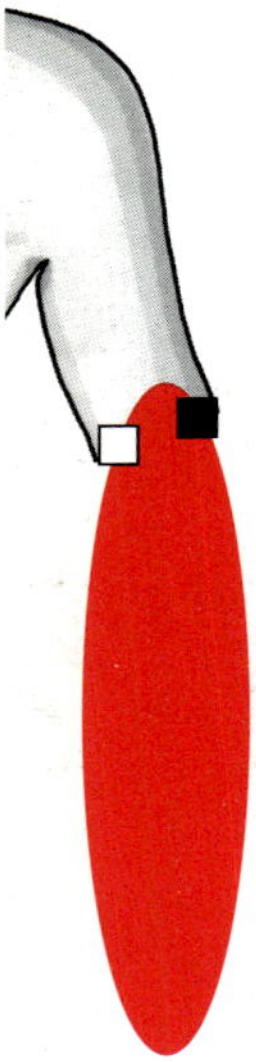

Inner aspect of arm

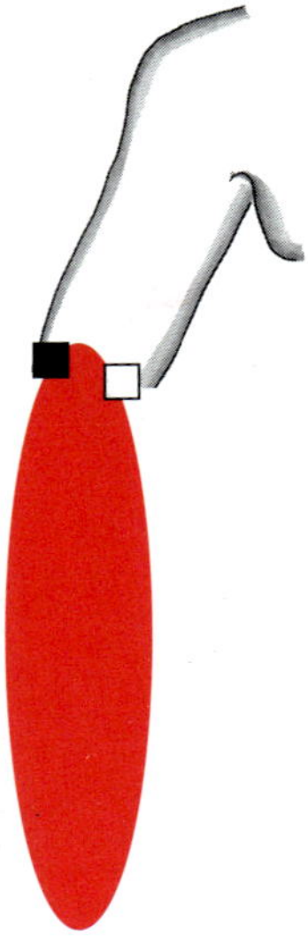

Phantom arm pain is shown by the red "pain zone". The black and white squares inside the "pain zone" represent two pairs of electrodes. Two electrodes are placed on the front of the arm and the other two on the back as shown in the diagrams. If you are using only one pair of electrodes, apply each pad centrally to the front and back of the stump.

Period pain or dysmenorrhoea

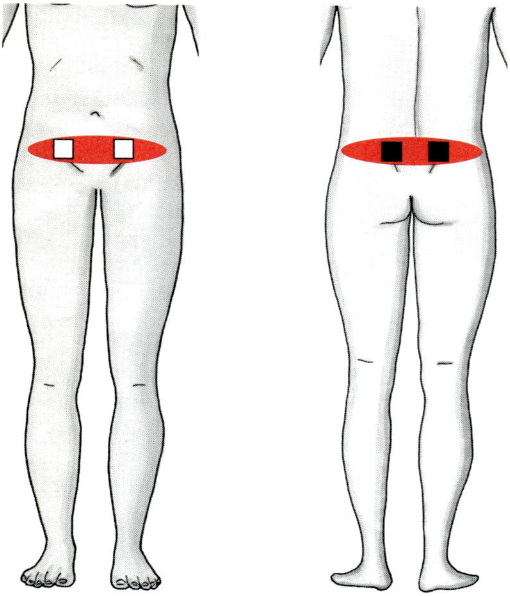

Period pain or dysmenorrhoea is shown by the red "pain zone". The black and white squares inside the "pain zone" represent two pairs of electrodes. One set of electrodes is placed on the front of the body and the other set is placed on the back of the body as shown in the diagrams.

Irritable bowel syndrome

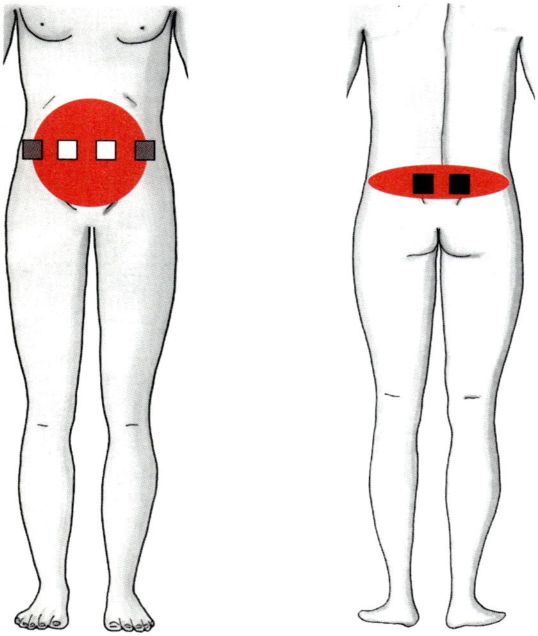

Irritable bowel syndrome is shown by the red "pain zone". The black and white squares inside the "pain zone" represent two pairs of electrodes. One set of electrodes is placed on the front of the body and the other set is placed on the back of the body as shown in the diagrams. The grey electrodes show an alternative placement position.

Classical migraine, headache, stress, Insomnia

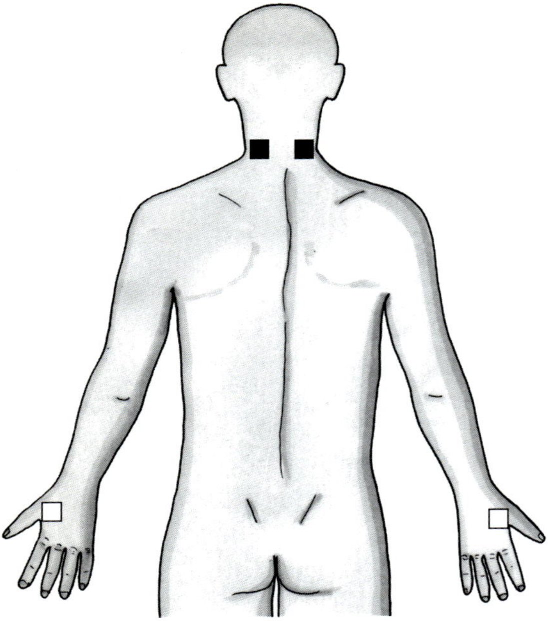

Classical migraine, headache, stress, insomnia are shown by the red "pain zone". The black and white squares represent two pairs of electrodes. The electrodes on the neck should border the hairline and be placed either side of the spine with 5cm (2″) between them.

The electrodes on the hands should be positioned on the web space between the first finger and thumb. If nausea and vomiting occur place electrodes on the inner arm 2.5cm (1″) from wrist crease.

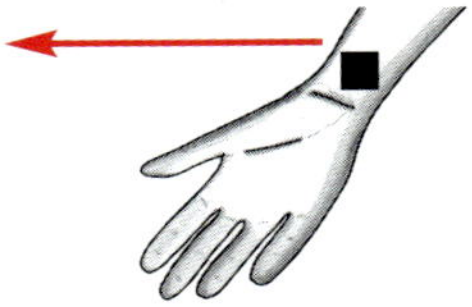

Pre-menstrual migraine and Tension (PMT)

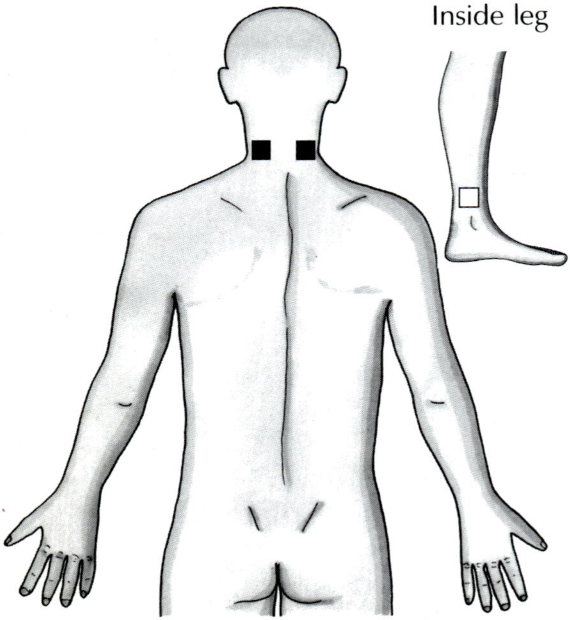

Inside leg

Pre-menstrual migraine and tension (PMT) are shown by the red "pain zone". The black and white squares represent two pairs of electrodes. The electrodes on the neck should border the hairline and be placed either side of the spine with 5cm (2″) between them.

One electrode should be placed on each inside leg as shown in the diagrams.

Trigeminal neuralgia

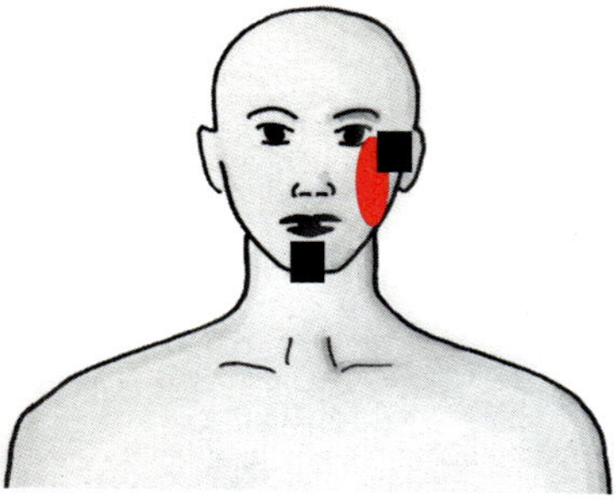

Trigeminal neuralgia pain is shown by the red "pain zone". The black squares represent a pair of electrodes. The electrodes are placed on the face as shown in the diagram. Stimulate very gently to begin with and stop if the pain worsens. Then try again, applying the electrodes to the opposite side of the face without the pain.

Post shingles (ophthalmic shingles) pain

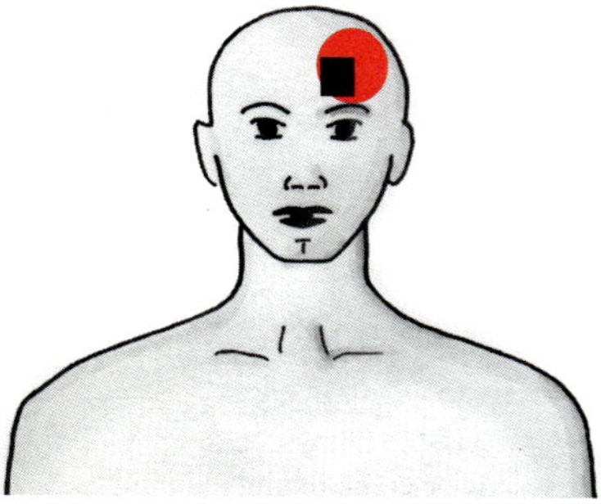

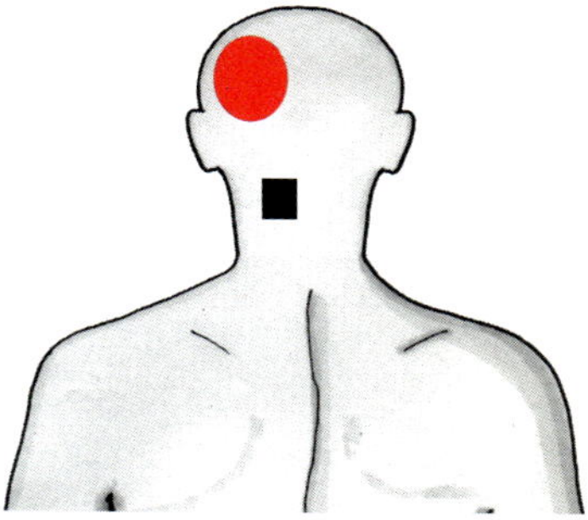

Post shingles ophthalmic pain is shown by the red "pain zone". The black squares represent a pair of electrodes. One electrode is placed on the forehead in the "pain zone", and the other on the back of the neck bordering the hairline as shown in the diagrams above.

Neuralgia Pain - Post shingles pain

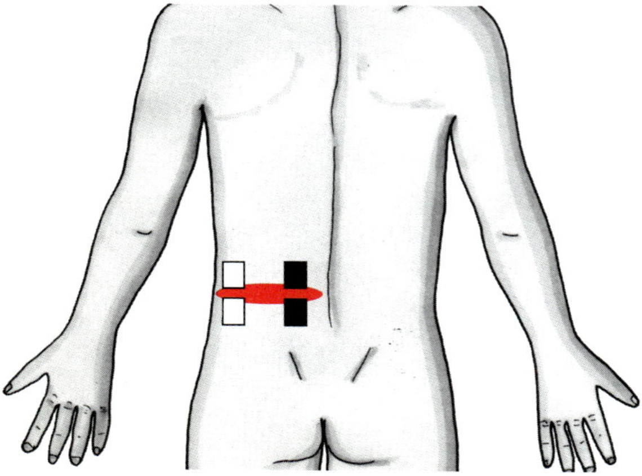

Post shingles pain is shown by the red "pain zone". The black and white squares inside the "pain zone" represent two pairs of electrodes. Place the electrodes on either side of the shingles scar wherever it is found on the body.

Post-operative neuralgia Chart 1

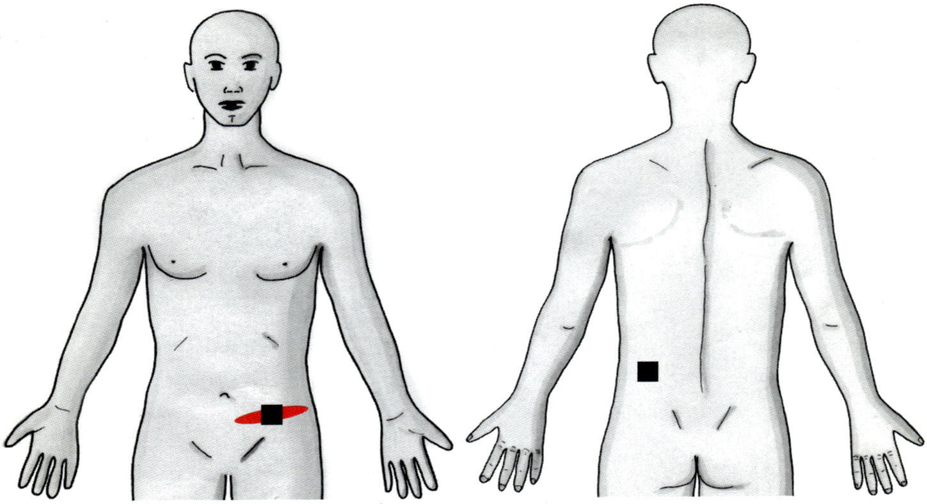

Post-operative neuralgia - An example is shown by the red "pain zone" but the scar could be sited anywhere on the body. One electrode should be placed over the scar and the other placed in the same position on the other side of the body, as shown in the diagrams above.

Post-operative neuralgia Chart 2

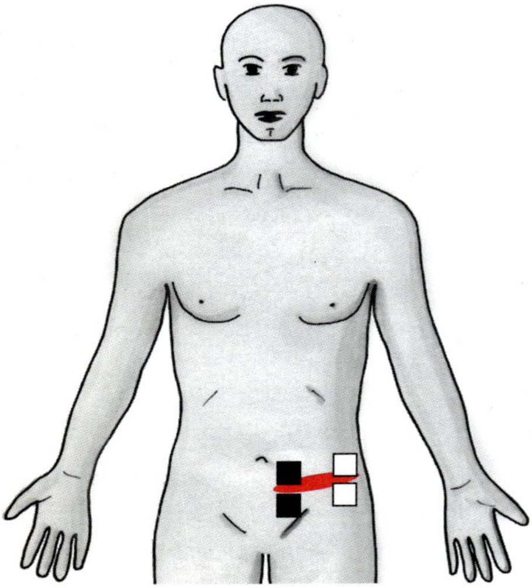

Post-operative neuralgia pain - The black and white squares inside the "pain zone" represent two pairs of electrodes. An example of how to treat this pain is shown but the scar could be sited anywhere on the body. The electrodes should be placed around the scar as shown in the diagram.

Nausea and vomiting associated with pregnancy, chemotherapy travel sickness, post operative, inner ear problems etc.

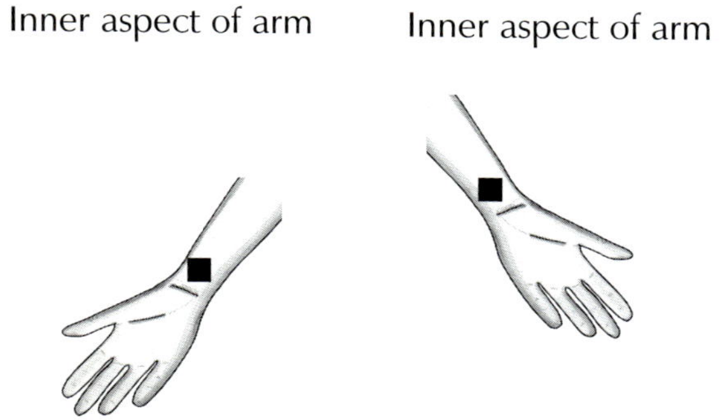

Nausea and vomiting. The black squares represent a pair of electrodes. Use a low frequency pulse rate for thirty minutes as needed. The electrodes should be placed on the inner aspect of both wrists, 2.5cm (1") from the wrist crease as shown.

Labour Pains

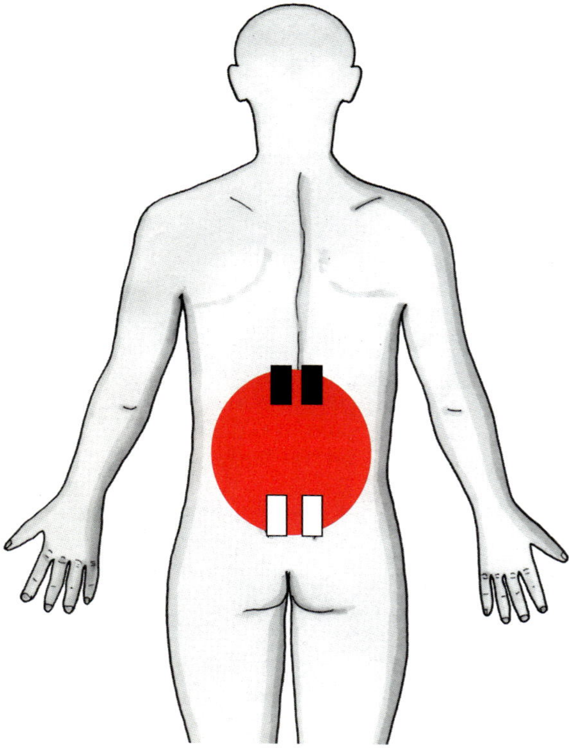

Labour and delivery - The black and white squares inside the "pain zone" represent two pairs of large obstetric electrodes. Place the electrodes on the lower back and mid back as shown in the diagram.

Please note that a Babycare TENS should be used for labour (supplied by Body Clock). These are specially designed units for childbirth.

Peripheral Neuropathy - associated with diabetes, chemotherapy, HIV etc

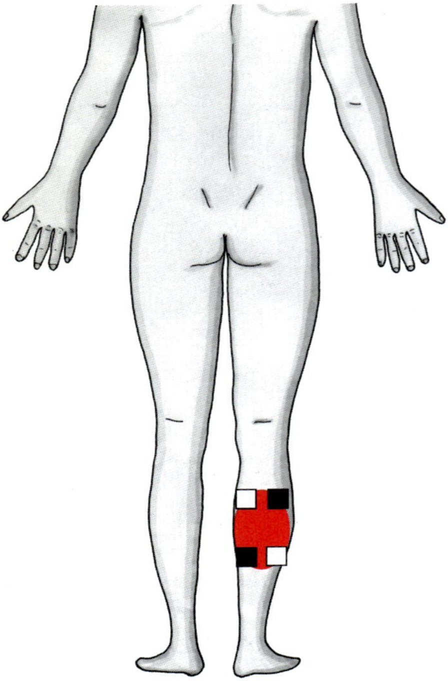

Peripheral Neuropathy The black and white squares inside the "pain zone" represent two pairs of electrodes. Place the electrodes on the leg as shown in the diagram.

Use a high frequency (pulse rate) and stimulate gently.

Wound/ulcer healing - associated with diabetes, varicose ulcer, post operative pain etc

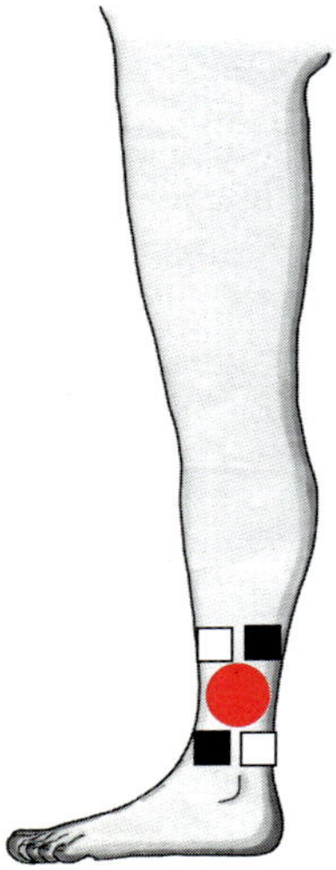

Wound/ulcer healing - The black and white squares inside the "pain zone" represent two pairs of electrodes. An example of how to treat this pain is shown, but the area of pain could be sited anywhere on the body.

Place electrodes surrounding the pain, not over broken or damaged skin. Use a high frequency (pulse rate) and stimulate gently.

III. A quick guide to setting up your TENS treatment

1. First - read this book and the "Instructions for Use" booklet which accompanies your Body Clock TENS.

2. Set up your unit in accordance with the "Instructions for Use" booklet.

3. Wash and dry around the area of pain, ensuring there is no grease or powder on your skin.

4. Apply self-adhesive electrodes to your skin. If using carbon rubber electrodes, use a small amount of gel and affix with surgical tape.

5. Make yourself comfortable for an hour or so while the treatment is working and re-read the instructions again until you are familiar with them. Take note of your pain level before the treatment. Try scoring the level of pain on a scale of 0-100, where 0 is no pain and 100 is the worst pain you have ever had. Record it on paper.

6. At the end of an hour switch the TENS unit off. If you want to begin treatment again within a few hours, you may leave the self-adhesive electrodes in position for the next treatment. If using non-adhesive electrodes remove them and wipe off the gel. Take note of your pain level now. Is it better or the same? Again, try scoring the level of pain on a scale of 0-100.

7. The next time you set up your TENS treatment it will be much easier. Deciding on the length of your next treatment, e.g 30mins, one hour or longer depends on the response you had with with your first treatment and whether you are going to rest or continue activities. You may wish to score the level of pain, before and after each treatment, as this will help to assess, over the next few days and weeks, how effective each treatment has been in reducing your pain level.

8. You may prefer to begin with just one treatment a day, or even three or four treatments, or use TENS continuously for a while depending on the severity of your pain.

9. You may then wish to adjust your TENS unit settings using a different mode, or different treatment times to gain more effective pain management, in line with the recommendations on page 24.

IV. How to use your TENS unit for pain management

TENS treatment can provide useful relief for both acute and chronic pain. TENS is self-administered, non-invasive and simple to use once you have mastered a few easy techniques.

General guidelines to help you manage your pain

1. Place electrodes over the painful area and stimulate. If this does not help then move the electrodes to either side of the pain, as shown on the Body Clock Electrode Placement Charts.

2. The sensation should feel comfortable. Low frequency TENS should produce a firm muscle twitching sensation. Your TENS unit must be set to a tolerable level.

3. As your TENS unit battery begins to drain, you may need to gradually increase the intensity to maintain the same level of stimulation output.

4. Research studies have shown that at least 30-60 minutes is needed for a conventional or burst mode TENS treatment to be effective. When using low frequency (acupuncture-like TENS) then 30 minutes is the recommended treatment time, which can be repeated after 90 minutes once or twice a day.

5. For "conventional" high frequency TENS there are no recommendations concerning total treatment time. Some find that short periods of 30-60 minutes can provide them with several hours of pain relief. Others find that they require longer treatment periods, perhaps for several hours or all day in order to achieve satisfactory pain relief.

6. Some patients find that one particular setting gives them the best pain relief. Others find it more comfortable to vary the settings. It is recommended that you consult your usual healthcare adviser to obtain the most effective pain relief advice. If this is not possible than this book will help you achieve the most effective response.

7. It is not usually recommended to use your Body Clock TENS during night time sleep, the reason being that if you roll over on to your electrodes, they may come off or be damaged.

8. All electrodes should be removed from the skin every day, and the surrounding area should be carefully washed and dried. Electrodes should not be applied to exactly the same area every day. Move them around slightly within the area of pain.

Do I need to take any special care of my skin?

1). TENS treatment produces very few side effects. Occasionally mild irritation at the electrode site may occur. This can usually be remedied by replacing the electrodes, gel or tape with alternative products.

2). When using carbon rubber electrodes and conductive gel, ensure the gel does not dry out. Add more if necessary to protect your skin.

3). Trim any excess body hair, which could interfere with smooth electrode contact with the skin, but do not shave it.

4). Do not place electrodes on cut, broken or irritated skin.

5). Moisturising cream may be applied after treatment, NOT before.

6). If irritation still occurs, discontinue use and consult your health care adviser.

Can I combine TENS with other therapies?

Yes - It can be combined with most other therapies such as conventional medication, physiotherapy, acupuncture, exercise, massage, homeopathy, herbal medicine, chiropractic and osteopathic manipulation, and hot and cold packs. However, if you have more than one treatment at a time, it may be difficult to know which treatment is helping you.

V. Are there any precautions to be taken with TENS?

Under which conditions should I not use a TENS unit?

1). Pain not diagnosed by your medical adviser.

2). If you have a demand-type cardiac pacemaker, serious or unstable heart condition or have had a recent heart attack.

3). Do NOT place electrodes on or near the eyes, in the mouth, over the front or sides of the neck, across the head, heart, or an area of broken, inflamed, infected, or numb skin. Electrodes should generally only be applied to skin with normal sensation unless under medical supervision.

4). Do not use TENS during pregnancy unless under medical supervision.

5). Do not use in the presence of tuberculosis, malignant tumours, very high or very low blood pressure, epilepsy, high fever or acute inflammatory disease unless under medical supervision.

6). If an allergic reaction develops to adhesive tape or electrodes.

7). If driving or operating potentially dangerous machinery.

8). Your TENS unit should be kept out of the reach of children.

9). Turn off your TENS unit while operating a microwave oven.

10). If you are in any doubt, contact your usual medical adviser.

VI. Routine maintenance

How do I care for, clean and store my TENS unit?
Your TENS unit requires no maintenance other than regular gentle cleaning. Using a soft cloth, slightly moistened with warm water, clean the case, leads and electrodes. A mild soap may also be used but DO NOT apply solvents.

Electrodes: Store self-adhesive electrodes in packaging provided in a cool, dry place. Follow instructions supplied to maintain adherence. Carbon rubber electrodes should be cleaned to remove conductive gel after use.

Batteries: The unit must be switched off when changing the battery.

TENS Leads: Do NOT yank or twist the leadwires - treat them gently for a long life. They are made from fine wire to be flexible and lightweight.

General Precautions.
Do not immerse your TENS unit in water or any other liquid
Do not place it close to any source of excess heat
Do not operate your unit in the presence of flammable gases
Do not attempt to open the TENS unit
Do not use battery or power sources other than those specified
Do not drop this unit onto a hard surface

Tell me about the Body Clock Warranty and Servicing
1). Body Clock TENS should be repaired by qualified technical personnel.

2). Body Clock TENS units are guaranteed for a period of 5 years against manufacturer's defects. Leads and carbon rubber electrodes are guaranteed for a period of three months.

3). Note: the guarantee is null and void if any attempt is made to open the unit by unauthorised personnel. In the event of a fault please contact Body Clock, 108 George Lane, South Woodford, E18 1AD. Tel: (+44) 020 8532 9595 Fax: (+44) 020 8532 9551 sales@bodyclock.co.uk

VII. Troubleshooting

If you are still having difficulty obtaining pain relief, carefully re-read this book and the "instructions for use" supplied. They contain all the information needed for success. Many people experience almost instant pain relief after following these instructions. Are you following all the instructions suggested? If so, and if you are still having difficulty in controlling your pain, try the following tips - one at a time.

1. You may need two or more treatments a day, sometimes for several hours, over several days. Even professionals do not always achieve instant relief for their patients: so do not abandon your TENS after just a few treatments. Continue use for two or more weeks at least, as the effects tend to be cumulative i.e. each treatment builds upon the last.

2. Experiment with different frequency settings bearing in mind the following guidelines:

(a) High pulse rate settings: Set the pulse rate above 10 and usually between 80-100 or more in continuous mode (C). This should be felt as a tingling sensation. Recommended treatment period is at least one hour, or for several hours continuously, for at least 2 or more weeks.

(b) Low pulse rate settings: Set the pulse rate below 10 and usually between 2-3 in continuous mode (C). This should be felt quite firmly. A treatment period of 30 minutes once or twice a day is usually sufficient once the pain is under control. You may also repeat the treatment 90 minutes later for an improved analgesic effect.

(c) Try pulse burst treatment (if this is available on your TENS model) by selecting B on your TENS and 100 on both the pulse rate and the pulse width for 30 minutes each treatment and repeat as required.

(d) If your TENS unit has an M setting (Pulse Modulation) then you can also try this setting again for 30 minutes each treatment, or longer if necessary. Some patients find this setting most helpful and soothing.

4. Make sure the electrodes are firmly in place at all times, in good condition and well-gelled. TENS electrodes are generally placed around the painful area, over the painful area, or over the acupuncture points in order to increase the effectiveness of TENS treatment.

5. If you are treating back pain try placing one electrode over the most painful area and the other on the opposite side of the spine. Also try placing the electrodes 2.5cm (1") either side of the spine, in line with the area of pain - i.e. 5cm (2") apart.

6. Try using different pulse rates during each treatment e.g 30 minutes on a high rate and 30 minutes on a low rate.

7. Try gently exercising the painful area while you are using your TENS unit and then applying a cold pack (from the fridge NOT out of the freezer) to the area for 10 minutes at the end of the treatment.

8. The most common cause of failure to achieve pain relief from TENS is too few treatments, so make sure you have given the treatment a really good trial and remember, the longer you have had your pain the longer it may take to reduce it and the more treatment you need.

9. Do not stop taking your usual pain killing drugs when you begin your pain treatment, but discuss reducing the dosage with your medical practitioner as your pain decreases.

10. Do not be afraid to experiment with different pulse rate settings to find the treatment which gives you the best result but give each change several days to work before switching to another one.

11. Enthusiastic tea or coffee drinking may reduce the analgesic effect of TENS - try cutting your intake down by half and drink water and fruit juices instead.

12. If your pain becomes worse, either during or after treatment, then it is usually due to applying the incorrect pulse rate for your problem. Try a different setting and if this does not help try moving the electrodes to another position and repeat until you achieve the pain relief you are looking for.

13. Remember: TENS treatment benefits most people but you have to give it a chance to work by ensuring an adequate trial i.e. treatments once or twice daily, or more, for at least 2-3 weeks, plus it may be necessary to adjust the pulse rate and/or the electrode placement to achieve the best effect.

Where can I find further supplies of accessories?
Call Body Clock Health Care on (+44) 020 8532 9595 for:- electrodes, batteries, gel, leads, sticky fixers, pouches, battery chargers and rechargeable batteries and much more, or order online at www.bodyclock.co.uk

What if I need more help?
Call us at Body Clock on (+44) **020 8532 9595** and we will do our best to assist.